POEMS

I0117865

By Isaac Hope

'One million people commit suicide every year'
The World Health Organization

Published by:
Chipmunkapublishing
PO Box 6872
Brentwood
Essex
CM13 1ZT
United Kingdom

http://www.chipmunkapublishing.com

Proof-read by Sofia Ribereiro

Cover Image by Simon Richardson

A Perfect Picture of Christmas

Santa flies the sky at night

Seeing him is a wonderful sight

With reindeer galloping across the sky

He stops in your house for a little mince pie

With a ring of the bell and a Ho ho ho

Santa rides through the falling snow

As in bed Children sleep

He brings them presents they'll love to keep

Santa flies the sky at night

Under the moon shinning bright

Santa clause with cheeks of red

Comes in your house when your tucked up in bed

He makes a day for you to remember

Brings warmth to the ice cold weather

He paints a perfect picture of Christmas

One that in pour hearts will last

He brings us seasonal joy

With a bottle of brandy or a nice new toy

An Angel's Moon

You're an Angel to me
The stars shine so you can see
As under the moon is where we sit
I think of how I'm so fortunate
For you I stop the tide
Fall from the sky, and glide
Don't know why
But you passed me by
Hope you come back soon
And we'll sit under another full moon

Angry Stormy Sea

Those grey clouds are here again
Though I'm like all other men
They always come and trouble me
And carry me out to sea
In the sea brews a mighty storm
As those grey clouds begin to form
The waves crash, bash and batter me
This angry stormy sea
But I'm strong and won't give in
If I have to I will swim
And am I going to get there
The land that's fine and fair
A land that's waiting for me
Right across this stormy sea

Bless The Possessed

The devil has made an abode of my head
At night he camps right under my bed
Salivates over the thought's of my mind
Red eyes peering at me from behind
Piercing my thoughts, piercing my brain
Putting me under a lot of strain
I sit here and suffer in silence
Feeling stressed feeling intense
I could easily break down and cry
For when I die I'm going to fry
Fry in a pan in the pits of hell
Suffocating on that nasty smell
So how do I redeem myself to the mighty God
But be poked by a red hot cattle prod
How do I prove to god my goodness
Will I ever be one for him to bless

Bullys

Seems everybody's picking on me

They all think it's so funny

Seems nobody likes me

Nobody want's to know me

They spit at me

Talk to me like a sting from a bee

Why am I not the same

Why do I always get the blame

Why do they never treat me the same

Why do they never want me to play in their games

Christmas Prayer

Christmas time is a time for a family reunion

A time for joy, happiness and love

A time to forget arguments and quibbles, stresses
and strains

A time to rejoice in the coming of the lord Jesus
Christ

Let us give thanks for his love and generosity

And remember the ones less fortunate

Invite them into our church and show them the
same love

and generosity the lord has shown us

Climb The Sea

Cities won't build themselves

And buckets won't dig wells

Goodnight mr insomniac

I'll see you when you wake up

Sailing a mountain peak

Climb the sea

Pick an apple from a pear tree

Creation

First there was God
And he was infinite
And souls dropped from him
Like apples from a tree
A soul wanted a body
His name was Adam
His body rose from pools of life
From his twelfth rib was given Eve
The human race thrived
Desire, the strongest of all evils
In the grip of desire
The race fought
Through war after war
But like ripples in the water
Someday to return to a state of bliss
And they shall return!

Daddy in the Navy

My dear old mommy
Used to tell me
That when I met my daddy
He would be big and strong
And no-more would anything ever go wrong
Because you see
My mommy
Met the perfect daddy
He's a hero in he navy
He's on a boat out at sea
But when he comes back to me
I will have the perfect family

Dear Beloved Granddad

You are the number one, bestest Granddad

Remembering you isn't sad

But I'm feeling blue

Because I can't be with you

Don't want to worry you, hope you don't mind

You were and are so kind

All I seemed to do

Was throw your love back at you

Maybe in the next life

Or the one after

We' be filled with laughter

Because the strife doesn't matter

We're only a world away

Though I feel I'm with you today

Don't ever forget me

I won't forget you

Take care Granddad

I love you man

Love from your Grandson

Demon Made of Flame

You demon voices
Sending messages to me
Making me quaking in my boots
But you never tell me
Why do you do this
Why do you do this to me
Sending me insane
Boiling blood in my brain
Again and again
I try to mend my membrane
But you won't be tame
You demon made of flame

Departed From The Membrane

Voices in my thoughts

Surfing the rivers of my mind

There's no way these animals will ever be tame

Wild beasts

There evilness never ceases

Cutting into my mind like a carving knife

Chopping it like a meat cleaver

Burning it with desires of ill

Take it all I pray

Take them away I pray

For years I've been saving you all from them

And I take all the damn blame

I'm not the same as I used to be

Used to think I was cool

That I'd grow up great

I'd be a top celebrity

But now I'm me

Angry

Insane

Departed from the membrane

Fucked up beyond belief, crazy

Save me!

<u>Despair in my Heart</u>

Sitting in a cage of darkness
Misery turns to despair
Despair leaps out
and leaves me here
Sitting a cage of darkness

Dog in Bloom

My family are to me
Compared to you
The highest mountain
To the deepest valley
Though I care for you
You enter my mind and cut it up
Make me to my family
The hungriest dog
With teeth so huge
To bite through wood
Though my heart is a flower in **bloom!**

Drink my way out of this

My insanity is pulling me down
I kick my feet around
Panic fight and kick
Sinking like a brick
The sinking sand has me stuck
No one gives a fuck
No one there with a rope
Or even a bicardi and coke
The sand is metaphoric
The drink'll get me bollocked
Still I want to drink it
And get the hell out of this **Shit!**

Environmental Scare

Help the future human race

Make haste, do not waste

Prevent worse conditions

With prohibitions, for high emissions

Stop making guns and bombs

Make right all our wrongs

There is no surplus, there is no spare

There is an environmental scare

Father and Son

Put Jesus Christ first
He's the ruler of the Universe
Comes from past the clouds
From high above
Riding on wings of love
Like a diamond clean and pure
Be faithful, be sure
Jesus we worship you
Because we know the Bible's true
Please oh please
Save us from our sinful deeds
God is there for everyone
God and Jesus Christ his son
So put your hands together and pray
Pray we will all have a better day

Feeling So Damn Blue

Loneliness creeps to my heart
I won't let it tear me apart
My heart yearns for a love that's true
To stop me feeling so damn blue

When I find a person
I get there and they've already gone
I could search the world that's wide
Sail the Ocean blue
Just to find someone who to me is true

Fire of Rage

Feeling so frustrated
I wanna burst with anger
The telly want's to suck me in
Chew on me like a piece of gristle
If I can I'll wriggle
Struggle, break free
Then what will I be
The same useless spineless
Weak punching bag
I wasn't always though
I used to argue punch and spit
Till I got locked up for it
I used to be an ever burning fire of rage
Then I changed my ways
Thought yeah I'll be tolerant, calm and resilient
Now I'm a stick of pink fluffy candy floss
Anyone's my boss
Till I snap, attack fight back
Or shall I crawl under a rock and die
Shall I not cry, but close my eye

Fade into the darkness, submit, give in

Suppose it's better than being an arrogant

Stuck up, fire of a fuck up

Gremlin

My mind is a gremlin
Spitting out thoughts in my mind
Feeding on my goodness
Feeding on my pride
My mind it has an ugly face
With all my thoughts out of place
Coming in, going out
Sometimes I don't know
What they're all about
Sometimes I sit there and want to shout
Sometimes I want to sit and cry
Sometimes I sit and watch my thoughts
Drifting slowly by

Guns or Food?

The government spends millions on killing
machines
But still their conscience gleams
It's not at all fair
To those without food out there
If I were blind would you steal from me
Would you let me be in poverty
If I were deaf would you talk behind my back
Or would you give me the things I lack
How can you afford an expensive pair of wheels
When millions go without meals
Do you know what's up their street
Not a beemer but something to eat
Do you ever think
About those who have nothing to drink
Sure as long as your alright
We will all sleep well tonight

He Loves Us All

Jesus Christ is the best
And he's the mightiest
Against evil he always wins
Saves us from our sins
Remember to repent
For Gods son he sent
Will save us all
Creatures great and small
Jesus christ is the king
With all the love he shall bring
He loves us all, his children
Won't judge people by the colour of our skin
For jesus is not a person of ruin
Nor is he the ruin of a person

Holy Christmas

Christmas time is a wonderful thing

The day that did Jesus bring

Open your hearts and we all sing

Honour to the greatest king

To remember the day of the birth of Christ

Celebrate Jesus and whilst

Remembering the three wise men

We give gifts like them

To the lord in highest above

Thank you for your support and love

This is the day that we remember

Jesus Christ, god's son the saviour

We pray for your divine love

We pray with the saints and angels above

We pray that one day women and men

Will live in peace on Earth again

Homeless at Christmas

I'm young and homeless and sitting in the street
I sit here and pray, you'll drop money at my feet
Remember me on Christmas day
I'm that homeless kid sitting in the street
Christmas time is a time to feel merry
Please remember, don't forget me
The festive season's just begun
But for me it's not all that fun
Sipping wine and feeling fine
Enjoying your families company all the time
To you a turkey is just a meal
To me it is a feast
Raining hard upon my head
How I wish I was snuggled up in bed
Every day is miserable for me
I'm desperate, or can't you see
All the Children with smiles wide
Tucked up warm and dry inside
The magic of Christmas has just begun
Looking forward to a season of fun

Who am I to complain

When I'm cold and wet and sitting in the rain

Just because I sleep in a park

And wake up all alone in the dark

What I'd give for a loaf of bread

What I'd give for a soft warm bed

What I'd give it must be said

To not be sitting on this cold wet street

Inside My Mind

Outside it's beautiful
Outside it's pretty
Inside my mind it's pretty shitty
This day's been good
This day's been bad
This day's been rather fucking mad
Yes I'm happy
Yes I'm glad
Inside my mind is dark and bad
No I'm not lonely
No I'm not sad
But yes I am rather mad

Iron Cage to Bliss

I'm trapped inside an iron cage
Taunted by a fiery rage
Mind in pieces
Torment never ceases
Complications overcome my mind
Evil of every kind
Wanting me to fall
To fall to my knees
I beg God please
Please save me from this
Take me to a higher bliss

Iron love

It's all about expression

The express train rides again

The huge iron beast rides out of my mouth

And into your heart

Badum badum

Beats the blood oxygenating organ

Whoo whoo

The whistle of the train

Ride on ride on

Iron machine

Irresistible Urges

Urges so irresistible

They wreak you

Tear you apart

Sink their teeth into your flesh

Frustration beyond reason

Burning thoughts

Hacking up vomit

Go away demons

Feeling of victory

One demon approaches

Now two, three

Victory gone

Smirking faces

Violent psychology

Urges to punch, smash, bash, pulverise

Go away demons

Go away!

Jolly Old Mr Christmas

Santa won't be coming this Christmas
'cos the dear old fella's out on the piss
He does want to he'll insist
This jolly old Mr Christmas

Every year he does his chore
Comes in your house just to hear you snore
He really is a good old bloke
Now he's left the pub and he's totally broke

He brought you socks the very last year
Now he's spent all his money on beer
A bit of gratitude would be great
The odd thank you he'd appreciate

So Santa won't be coming this Christmas
Cos the dear old fella's out on the piss
He does want to he'll insist
This jolly old Mr Christmas

Joy In My Soul

God's love goes deep into the soul

God's love is whole

For the age of time

God is divine

I crave for love everyday

I sit and pray

God will you rescue me, my mortal soul

But will he let me fall

Or will he help me swim against the tide

Will he let me walk with pride

Maybe not, maybe so

Is he friend or is he foe

Will he in my soul

Allow joy to grow

Just The Way I Feel

Loneliness like a dark depressing cloud
A thick layer of despair
No rain, or water to drink
No sun to melt the ice
No way out of this torment
Just stress and frustration to put me deeper
Up the proverbial shit creek
Without the proverbial paddle
I'm deep under water
It's a long way down
I'm going to fall
I'm going to drown

Lion's Despair

Here I am in the murky waters of despair

Don't know why I'm just there

Floating in the black waters of depression

All my sanity has just gone

This diamond has a kink in the side

This lion has lost his pride

I'm six feet under

When I wonder

What's it like up there

Is the sun shinning bright

Is there a full moon at night

If I just reach the top

Will this sadness finally stop

Love Fatigue

Is there any love in me
Do I have a love fatigue
Are my emotions full of water
Is love an emotional torture
If you don't have any love
Can you ascend to the world above
If your heart is full of hate
Will you reach Heavens gate
If your heart is black as coal
Will there be love in your soul
If all you care about in life
Is all your money and all your strife
Can your life ever be **suffice!**

Love Hater

I'm a love hater
Love makes me sick
Love makes me want to attack it
Beat it with a stick
Love has broken my heart in two
Left me gormless, without a clue
Love is a knife stuck in my chest
Anyone in love, they should arrest
Love is beautiful
Love is gold
Love is everything
Or so I'm told

Love Overcomes The Tsunami

Disaster, disaster struck this world again
When will this world ever be tame
When will this world give us love
Will happiness rain down from above

Terror creeps into our hearts
As a wave destroys these eastern parts
Bodies swept far and wide
By a hungry, and angry tide

Waves rip through the land of the rising sun
As our governments spend another dollar on a
gun
A dollar, a dollar on a meal
An autograph on a peace deal

Sometimes all people can do or say
Is beg God in a word of pray
On this devastating Christmas hour
All our prayers must have turned sour

Sometimes the rain pours down on me
Sometimes the wind blows down a tree
Sometimes the sun shines high and bright
Sometimes it rains right through the night

Help these people
Help them through
Do the best that you can do
Do it because they depend 0n you

Disaster, disaster
Once more we've overcome
Maybe today the fight we have won
Maybe today our hearts will fill with love as one.

Madness to Peace

My mind was in pieces
Now it's back together
All the symptoms of schizophrenia
Changing like the weather
Now peace is upon my soul
And my mind's together now it's whole
With a strong sense of direction
I know I'll achieve
When I express myself
this is what I believe

Mental Torment

Crushed in mental torment

Can the heart speak

Or is it too weak

One more spliff

One more cigarette

One more pint of beer and I'll forget

Money and Wealth

You cannot buy the stars

You cannot buy the sea

And will money really fill you with glee

Will it make you happy

Can a piece of paper make you a king

Can paper make you sing

Can it bring the best of life

Can it save you from a knife

Will it bring the love of your child

Will it kill a lion in the wild

Will it make you prince of pop

But then again

Will it make your heart just

Stop!

My Red Dead Eyes

My body weakens

My heart is pumping

My pen is speaking

My nerves are jumping

My anger turns to rage

As I look at the walls of my cage

I see red

I don't fight, no instead

I close my eyes

I start to cry

And wish to die

Not Grace Nor Love

Inside my heart
Is a lonely place
Inside my mind there is no grace
Inside my soul
I have no friends
Inside my life
All bitter ends

Poetic Christmas

Capture a twinkle in a little ones eyes
Brandy butter on mince pies
A little blue present with a bright red bow
Brought by a man who flew through the snow
Kisses under the mistletoe
The smell of chestnuts on the stove
In the light of the old log fire
Stands a local Christian choir
With a blanket of snow on the outside floor
And a holy reef on the front door
Santa flies above the ground
As snow falls without a sound
A chubby man with cheeks of rose
And a flying reindeer with a bright red nose

Poison Mind

Poison thoughts bite into my mind

As I squirm and wriggle inside

Then they sink their teeth right in

A nail enters into my skin

Like that of a voodoo doll

I try to escape, try to scale the wall

But the wall's too high

If I stay, I die

Begging god for some support

But he says freedom won't be bought

So I ask an Angel

She says I belong in hell

So what do I do with this illness

Hopw do I stop being oppressed

So here I am, and what I say

Is all a word of pray

I'm not a bad man

Don't want to be

That's just how I am

Little old me

Robin Redbreast

Little robin redbreast
Only comes round here at Christmas
A soft white blanket made of snow
Falling gently outside my window
Chestnuts roasting on an open fire
On the doorstep stands a singing choir
A picturesque blanket lays outside
As we warm by the fire dry inside
Little robin sing out loud
Sitting under a snowing cloud
A snow man made of glistening snow
With a nice pink and yellow pocodot bow
Outside where the children play
Sliding down hills on a wooden sleigh
Decorations hanging from the ceiling
Bobble on the tree glistening, gleeming

Rotten to the Core

Bleeding out lyrics from the pours of my skin
Something's rotten to the core from deep within
Rotten to the core from deep within
Rotten to the core from deep within
As my heart starts splitting as I begin To sing
No point knocking 'cos no-ones in
This cracked up mind's in the loony bin
Yeah I'm sitting in a loony bin
Yeah I'm sitting in the loony bin
This is the soul that you're killing
The drugs make my mind keep spinning
I die as this song is fin-ish-ing.

Savage Beasts

There's a pack of hyenas
hunting me down
They roam around
Filthy savage beasts
Prey on the weak
Like ghosts in the night
For scraps they fight
They want to eat the flesh of me
Wrestle me to the mud with their teeth
They'll drain my blood
for a thirsty feast
just to prove they can
and
they spot me with an evil eye
in the night they howl and cry
because their hunger will never cease
they're searching for another meal
just one more giant feast

<u>Shine Through the Evilness</u>

Evil thoughts stacked on my head

Gonna break through my skull like a tone of lead

Poison my thoughts poison my mind

Poison my tattered soul inside

Just when is the light going to break through

Who will I be and what will I do

I'll sit here all on my own

And speak to you in a tortured tone

<u>Skydiving Love</u>

Your love is like a dove

So pure and white it flies above

Your love is like a skydive

On your love the food I thrive

So sing with me

Love me purely, completely, fantastically

I love you valentine

Say I'm yours, say you're mine

Loving you is no crime

Loving you is a love sublime

Your face of delight

Is such a gracious sight

Our hearts are much the same

We belong to together like picture and frame

Snowdrop Tears

I cannot cry
Though tears are welling in my eye
Behind a barrier in my mind
The saddest sadness you'll ever find
One day it will come
the tears will start to run
then not he best of things
will ever stop the flow
it will run through summer
then in winter, it will fall as snow

<u>Technicality</u>

My mind has a technicality

With thoughts as calm as a stormy sea

Sometimes they are black

Sometimes they are white

They dent my ego

They dent my pride

Sometimes they come

Sometimes they hide

Sometimes they destroy everything inside

Telepathy

My mind feels open
People peering in
Looking at my mind
For a memory of sin
My mind is public property
Or so they fucking think
For once I tried to drown myself
In the fucking sink
Thought the world was doomed
My fault it must have been
But then, to save the world
I-am-always-keen

The Day Today

Death suspense

Alien defence

Guns, bombs

Playtex condoms

Elicit drugs

Wild thugs

Rap songs

Glass bongs

High emissions

Harsh conditions

Committing crime

Doing time

Designer vests

Police arrests

Clever computers

Small flat

Tabby cat

Waste time with another useless rhyme

The Robot Named Stan

One day he will come
The battery eating electric bum
A standard man named Stan
Not a black, white or yellow man
But an aluminium chunk of metal
An evolutionized electric kettle

The Tree of Life

Once I thought there was something here
Something to entertain us in this lost world
Drifting through space, drifting through time
Existing only to keep the population up
To please our God and Buddha
Doing the right things, But for what?
Who notices?
I've been staring at commodities for years
Only to be discontented by their existence
Desire.
To become empty and useless,
As soon as the desire is fulfilled
To enter existence we beat thousands of
contenders
In the race to the mighty ova
Everyday beating overwhelming odds
To stay alive, only to prolong death.
And whither and die like a leaf in autumn
But when we're gone the tree still stands
Did it notice we were there?

Has it noticed we're gone?

The Universe

Where are we, what are we

We are six billion men and women

Made of many more number of atoms

On a rock, orbiting a star we call the sun

Belonging to a solar system

Cascading through dark space

Surrounded by a phenomenally large universe

So small it fits inside an atom of a higher state

As a building block o0f a much larger world

Which may or may not be inhabited

Maybe Heaven, maybe hell

To build this gigantic world

Billions of trillions of other atoms

Inside them Universes dark and light

With galexes all shapes and sizes

Made of planets of all colours

And races of men and women, all fighting for life

All trying to do the best thing

Cascading through darkness

Saying to each other

where are we, what are we.

The Word of God

In this world there is one word
That is the word of God
The lord is the greatest king
Across the world people sing
Sing about the love he's bringing
Don't you sin against the lord
For that is breaking the word of God

Too Late

My mind is broken

My mind's not the same

My mind's been hit by a runaway train

My mind is derelict

My mind's a mess

Fuelled more and more by an intense stress

My mind's complicated

My mind's irate

And I think, to save me, you're a little too late

Wave of Destruction

The sound I hear
Fills me with fear
Then I see
The tsunami
Comes rolling in
Destroying everything
People screaming is it real
So many that wave did kill
A giant wave of water
As I'm bathing in the sun
The tsunami came and ruined all my fun
A minute later thousands are dead
Thousands screaming
Is it real, am I dreaming
All this carnage
From a raging wave
All there people no-one did save

Who's in the Mirror

I'm a very different person to who I thought I was
I'm a very different person to who I thought I'd be
I'm drowning in my sorrow
Like drowning out at sea
When I look in the mirror in the morning
Who do I think I am
But someone looking in the mirror
Wondering who I think I am

Wild Heartless Tiger

Tiger wild, tiger within

Tiger fire in my eyes

A tiger wild in my heart

A tiger I through death depart

Tiger fearless

Tiger ferocious

Tiger dead lying motionless

Wolf

Trapped
Standing in a corner
Back against the wall
I'm tiny
And he's ten feet tall
A wolf
Blood dripping from his teeth
I show fear in my eye
He breaths a hungry sigh
Then he pounces
With a leap toward me
He's a killer with a taste for me
Flesh is what he want's
And death is what he get's
When I grab a knife
And stick it in his chest

www.ingramcontent.com/pod-product-compliance
Lightning Source LLC
Chambersburg PA
CBHW031140270326
41931CB00007B/631